Gout Friendly Recipes

A Cookbook to Get You Through the Diets If You Have Gout

By

Angel Burns

© 2019 Angel Burns, All Rights Reserved.

License Notices

This book or parts thereof might not be reproduced in any format for personal or commercial use without the written permission of the author. Possession and distribution of this book by any means without said permission is prohibited by law.

All content is for entertainment purposes and the author accepts no responsibility for any damages, commercially or personally, caused by following the content.

Get Your Daily Deals Here!

Free books on me! Subscribe now to receive free and discounted books directly to your email. This means you will always have choices of your next book from the comfort of your own home and a reminder email will pop up a few days beforehand, so you never miss out! Every day, free books will make their way into your inbox and all you need to do is choose what you want.

What could be better than that?

Fill out the box below to get started on this amazing offer and start receiving your daily deals right away!

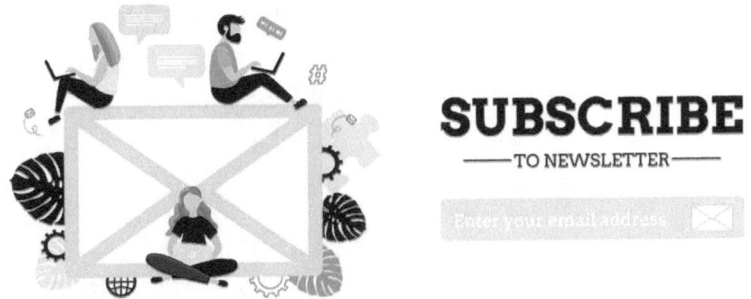

https://angel-burns.gr8.com

Table of Contents

Simple Gout Friendly Recipes 7

    Recipe 1: Green Bean Chowder 8

    Recipe 2: Zucchini Crab Cakes 11

    Recipe 3: Roasted Kabocha Squash 13

    Recipe 4: Braised Balsamic Chicken 15

    Recipe 5: Watermelon Juice 18

    Recipe 6: Slow – Cooker Vegetarian Chili 20

    Recipe 7: Turmeric & Pineapple Juice 22

    Recipe 8: Rosemary Watermelon Lemonade 24

    Recipe 9: Curried Fish 26

    Recipe 10: Salsa Chicken Burritos 29

    Recipe 11: Cherry, Banana & Strawberry Smoothie 31

    Recipe 12: Lemon Dill Salmon 33

    Recipe 13: Brown Stewed Chicken 35

Recipe 14: Potato and Vegetable Frittata 38

Recipe 15: Creamy Peanut Soup 41

Recipe 16: Honey Mustard Chicken 43

Recipe 17: Lentil Soup 46

Recipe 18: Vanilla Fruit Salad 48

Recipe 19: Spicy Pan-Fried Chicken 50

Recipe 20: Slow Cooker Chicken Stew 52

Recipe 21: Hoisin Chicken Filled Lettuce Wraps 54

Recipe 22: Cherry Smoothie 56

Recipe 23: Sweet & Spicy Chicken Wings 58

Recipe 24: Mushroom & Chicken Stuffed Bell Peppers 61

Recipe 25: Grilled Chicken & Green Bean Salad 64

Recipe 26: Chicken Mince Salad 66

Recipe 27: Garlic Mashed Red Potato 69

Recipe 28: Roasted Carrot & Bell Pepper Soup 71

Recipe 29: Sunomono Salad 74

Recipe 30: Sweet & Nutty Fruit Salad 76

About the Author 78

Author's Afterthoughts 80

Simple Gout Friendly Recipes

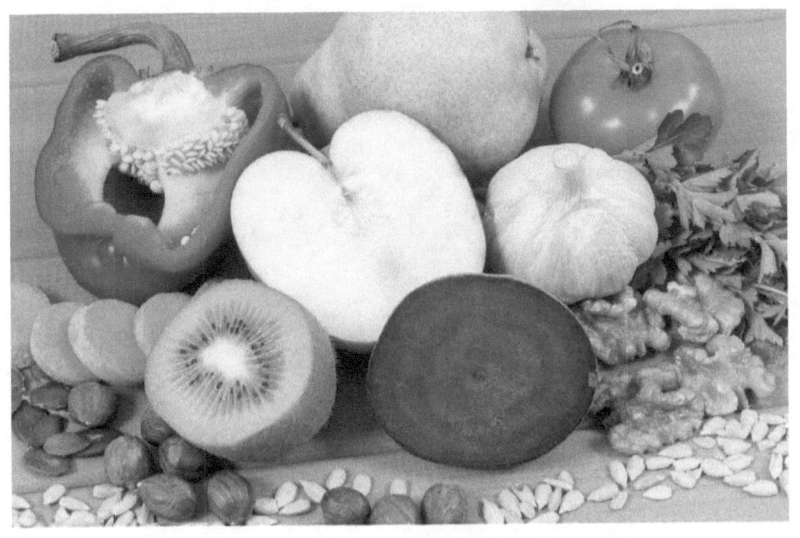

HHHHHHHHHHHHHHHHHHHHHHHHHHHHHHHHHHH

Recipe 1: Green Bean Chowder

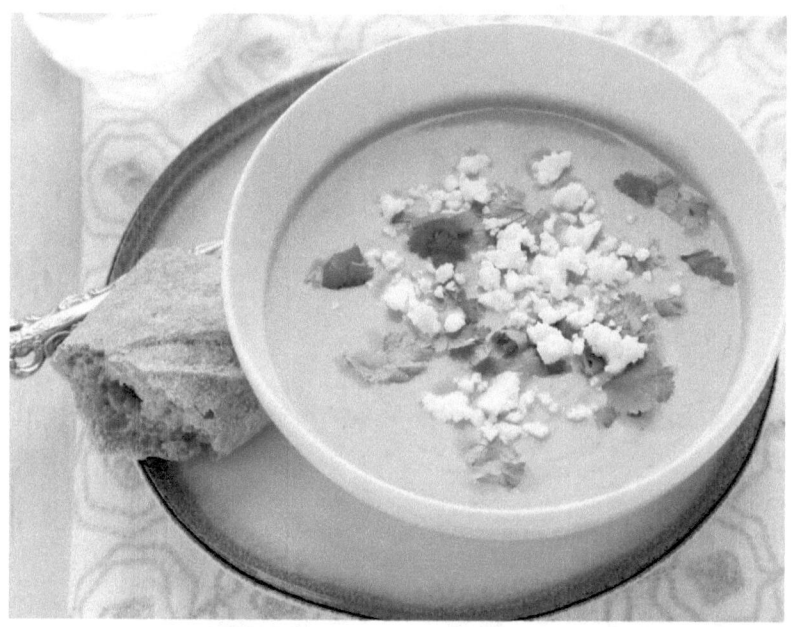

Beans are a valuable source of proteins and when used in a chowder you get to enjoy all these benefits in every bite.

Yield: 4

Preparation Time: 5 hours 30 minutes

Ingredient List:

- 1 cup green beans
- 14oz. can coconut milk
- 1 cup water
- 1 ½ tablespoon yellow curry paste
- 3 garlic cloves, minced
- ¼ cup orange juice
- ½ cup diced tomatoes
- ½ cup diced potatoes
- 1 tablespoon dried parsley
- ¼ teaspoon fresh thyme
- 1 tablespoon minced ginger
- 2 teaspoons sugar
- 1 teaspoon hot sauce
- Salt and pepper- to taste

HHHHHHHHHHHHHHHHHHHHHHHHHHHHHHHH

Instructions:

1. Place green beans in the slow cooker.

2. Add the garlic, potatoes, ginger, sugar, hot sauce, and curry paste.

3. Pour the orange juice and water.

4. Cover and cook on high for 4-5 hours.

5. Add the remaining ingredients and cook for 20 minutes more.

6. Serve while still hot.

Recipe 2: Zucchini Crab Cakes

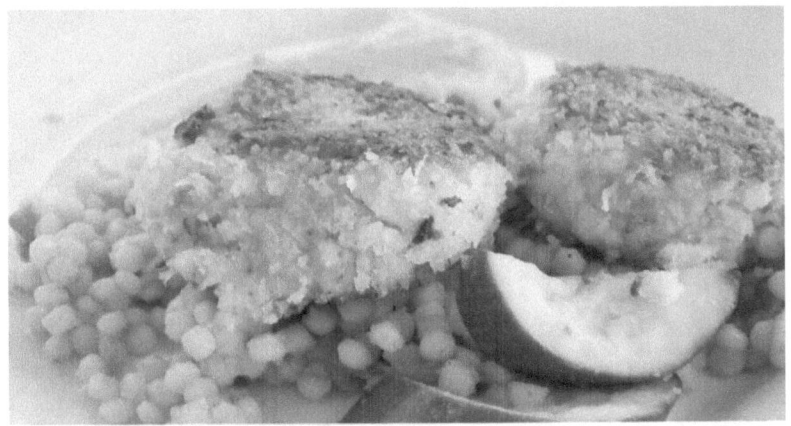

You don't need crab to enjoy delicious crab cakes. Now you can enjoy the same amazing feeling using zucchini.

Yield: 6

Preparation Time: 30 minutes

Ingredient List:

- zucchini (2 ½ cups, grated)
- egg (1, beaten)
- butter (2 tablespoons)
- Breadcrumbs (1 cup)
- onion (¼ cup, minced)
- Old Bay Seasoning (1 teaspoon)
- Flour (¼ cup)
- vegetable oil (½ cup, to be used for flying)

HHHHHHHHHHHHHHHHHHHHHHHHHHHHHHHHH

Instructions:

1. Combine all your ingredients, except oil and flour, in a large bowl and mix well.

2. Shape your mixture into 12 even patties, and dredge in flour.

3. Set a skillet over medium heat, add your oil and allow to get hot.

4. Fry your patties until perfectly golden on both sides.

5. Serve and enjoy.

Recipe 3: Roasted Kabocha Squash

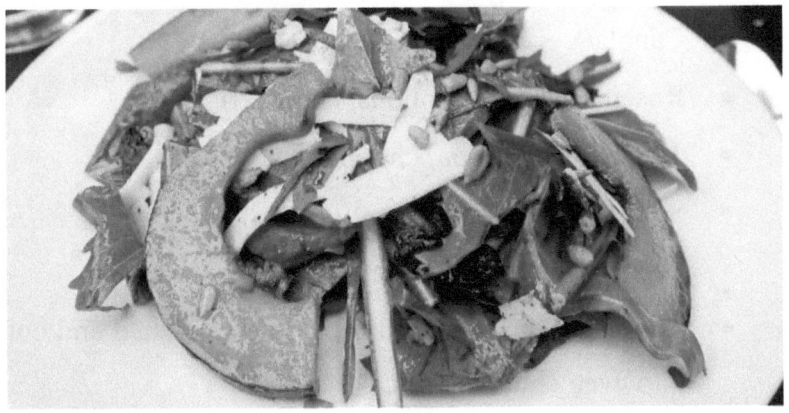

Kabocha squash is mildly sweet in flavor but tends to go well with just about any protein as a side, or on its own as a snack.

Yield: 4

Preparation Time: 35 minutes

Ingredient List:

- Onion (1 small, chopped)
- Canola/Vegetable Oil (2 tablespoons)
- Rosemary (2 tablespoons, chopped)
- Thyme (1 teaspoon, chopped)
- Salt (¼ teaspoons)
- Pepper (1/8 teaspoons)
- Kabocha Squash (1 ½ lbs., skin on, washed and cut into even chunks)

HHHHHHHHHHHHHHHHHHHHHHHHHHHHHHHHH

Instructions:

1. Set your oven to preheat to 450 degrees F, and grease your baking sheet then set aside.

2. In a large bowl create a rub by mixing together your rosemary, salt, pepper, onion, thyme, and oil.

3. Throw in your squash and toss until well coated. Line a ¬layer of squash onto your baking sheet ensuring that none overlaps.

4. Bake until squash is tender and light brown in color.

5. Serve.

Recipe 4: Braised Balsamic Chicken

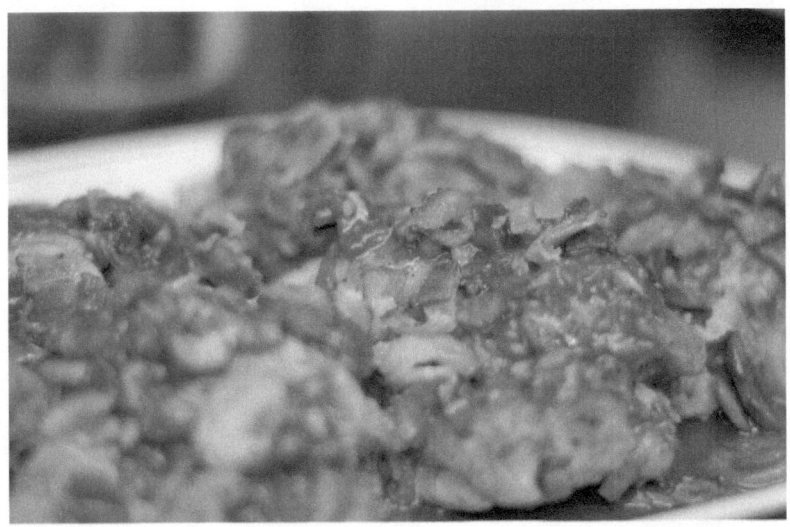

For a delicious low-fat, gout friendly dinner option be sure to try this Braised Balsamic Chicken.

Yield: 6

Preparation Time: 35 minutes

Ingredient List:

- chicken breast (6, skinless, halved)
- garlic salt (1 teaspoon)
- Black pepper (1 teaspoon)
- Olive oil (2 tablespoons)
- Onion (1, thinly sliced)
- tomatoes (14.5 ounces, diced)
- balsamic vinegar (½ cup)
- basil (1 teaspoon)
- oregano (1 teaspoon)
- Rosemary (1 teaspoon)
- thyme (½ teaspoons)

HHHHHHHHHHHHHHHHHHHHHHHHHHHHHHHHHH

Instructions:

1. Use your garlic salt and pepper to lightly seasoned chicken breast and sets aside.

2. In a skillet, heat your olive oil over medium heat.

3. Next, add in your chicken then allow to cook until perfectly browned (about 4 minutes on each site).

4. Next, add onions and cook until fragrant (about another 4 minutes).

5. Add the remaining ingredients, and allows a similar until fully cooked (about another 15 minutes, the chicken should have an internal temp. of at least 165° F). Enjoy!

Recipe 5: Watermelon Juice

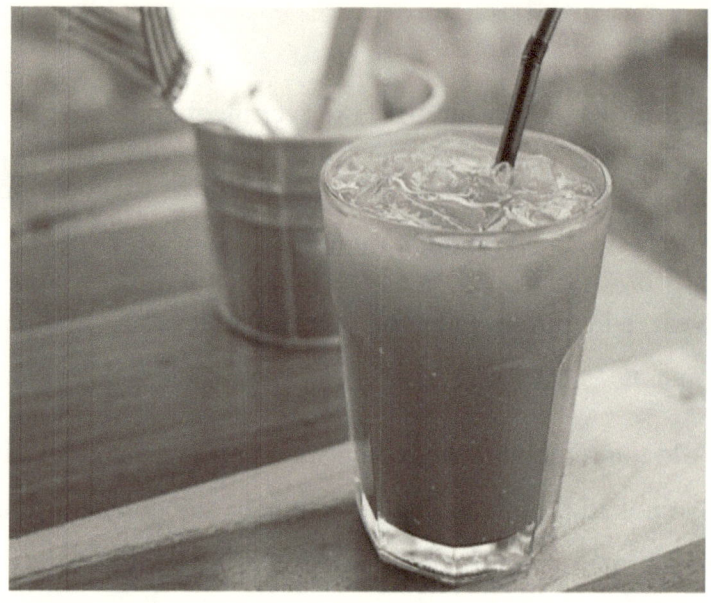

Watermelon is good for gout as it has a high water content, and water is great for flushing out your system.

Yield: 1

Preparation Time: 5 minutes

Ingredient List:

- 1 cup watermelon (seeds removed, and diced)
- 1 dash stevia powder
- 1 cup water

HHHHHHHHHHHHHHHHHHHHHHHHHHHHHHHH

Instructions:

1. In a blender add all ingredients and blend well.

2. Serve and enjoy.

Recipe 6: Slow – Cooker Vegetarian Chili

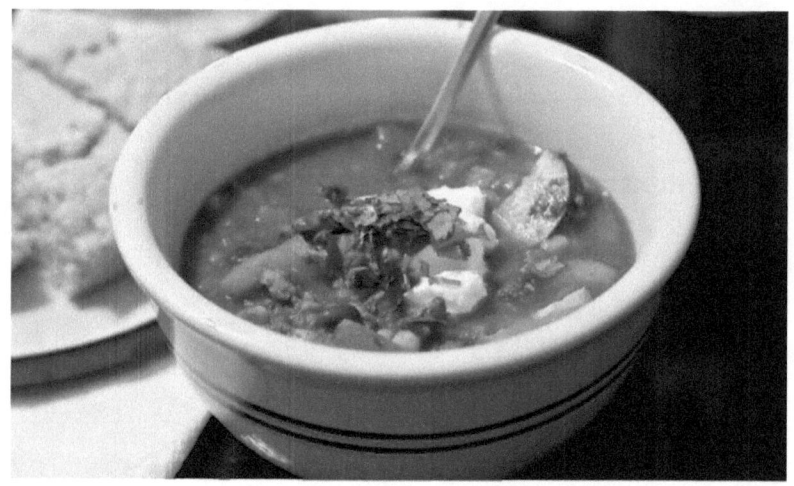

Now you can enjoy gout friendly twist off delicious gout friendly chili.

Yield: 8

Preparation Time: 2 hours 15 minutes

Ingredient List:

- Black bean soup (19 ounces)
- Kidney beans (15 ounces)
- Garbanzo beans (15 ounces)
- Baked beans (16 ounces, vegetarian)
- Tomatoes (14.5 ounces, canned, puréed)
- Corn (15 ounces)
- Onion (1, chopped)
- Bell Pepper (1, Green, chopped)
- Celery (2 stalks, chopped)
- Garlic (2 cloves, minced)
- Chili powder (1 tablespoon)
- Parsley (1 tablespoon, dried)
- Oregano (1 tablespoon, dried)
- Basil (1 tablespoon, dried)

HHHHHHHHHHHHHHHHHHHHHHHHHHHHHHHH

Instructions:

1. Combine all your ingredients in a slow cooker, and allow to cook on high for about 2 hours. Enjoy!

Recipe 7: Turmeric & Pineapple Juice

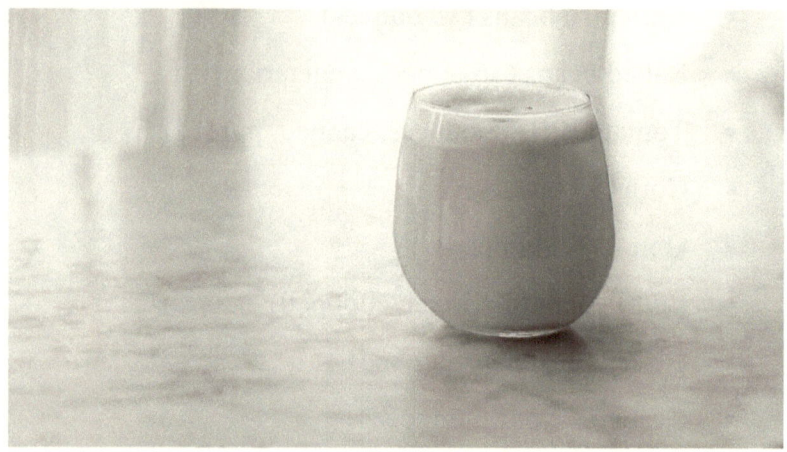

This mixture is rich in vitamin C and bromelain that are both great for reducing uric acid and relieving joint pain.

Yield: 1

Preparation Time: 5 minutes

Ingredient List:

- 1 cup pineapple (diced)
- 1 dash stevia powder
- 1 tablespoon turmeric
- 1 cup water

HHHHHHHHHHHHHHHHHHHHHHHHHHHHHHHH

Instructions:

1. In a blender add all ingredients and blend well.

2. Serve and enjoy.

Recipe 8: Rosemary Watermelon Lemonade

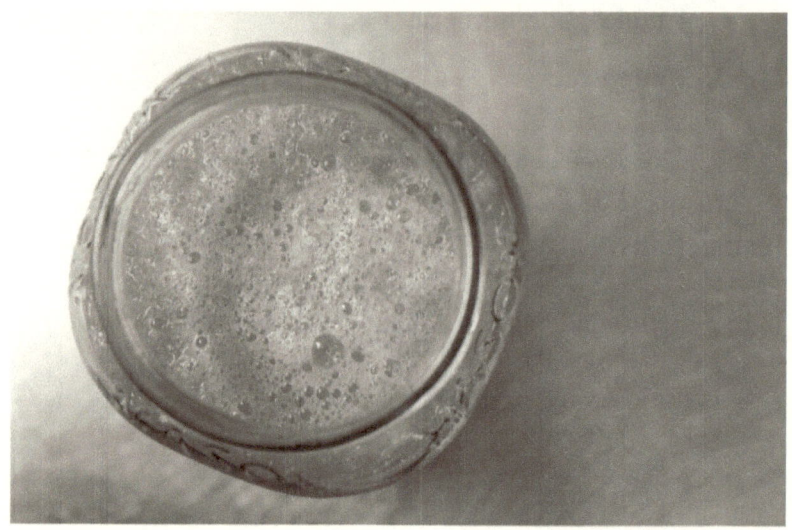

If you have trouble drinking water, this lemonade will be a good compromise.

Yield: 8

Preparation Time: 15 minutes + infusing time

Ingredient List:

- water (2 cups)
- sugar (¾ cup)
- Rosemary (1 sprig, leaves, chopped)
- lemon juice (2 cups)
- watermelon (12 cups, cubed)
- ice (8 cups)

HHHHHHHHHHHHHHHHHHHHHHHHHHHHHHHHH

Instructions:

1. In a medium saucepan, allow your water and sugar to come to a boil over high heat.

2. Once boiling, add your Rosemary, remove from heat, cover and allow to sit for at least an hour.

3. Strain your Rosemary syrup to remove rosemary leaves, then add all your ingredients to a blender.

4. Until smooth, strain, and serve over ice. Enjoy!

Recipe 9: Curried Fish

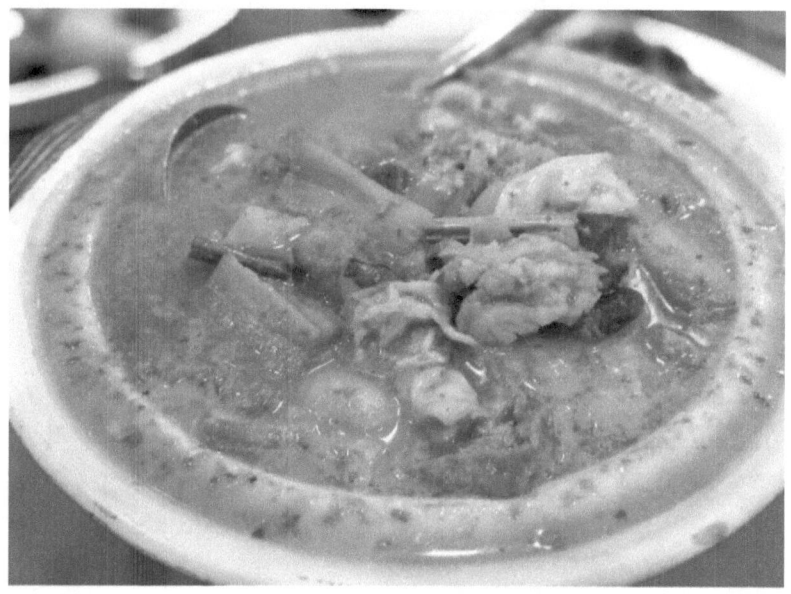

If you have never tried curried fish, then this may be the recipe for you.

Yield: 4

Preparation Time: 8 hours 10 minutes

Ingredient List:

- 1 teaspoon ground coriander seeds
- 2 tablespoons yellow curry paste
- 4 garlic cloves, minced
- 1 lb. cod, rinsed and dried then cubed
- ½ lb. green beans, cut into ½-inch pieces
- 1 cup finely chopped brown onion
- 4 small carrots, chopped
- 2 medium potatoes, cut into ½-inch slices
- ½ teaspoon cayenne pepper
- 1 ½ cup fish stock
- 1 cup coconut milk
- 1 teaspoon Fresh ground salt and pepper

HHHHHHHHHHHHHHHHHHHHHHHHHHHHHHHHH

Instructions:

1. Add your curry in a saucepan with oil over medium heat, and cook until fragrant (about a minute).

2. Add in your fish and allow to lightly brown in curry for about 2 minutes per side.

3. Combine all your remaining ingredients.

4. Cover and cook on medium for 20 minutes.

5. Season to taste, serve, and enjoy.

Recipe 10: Salsa Chicken Burritos

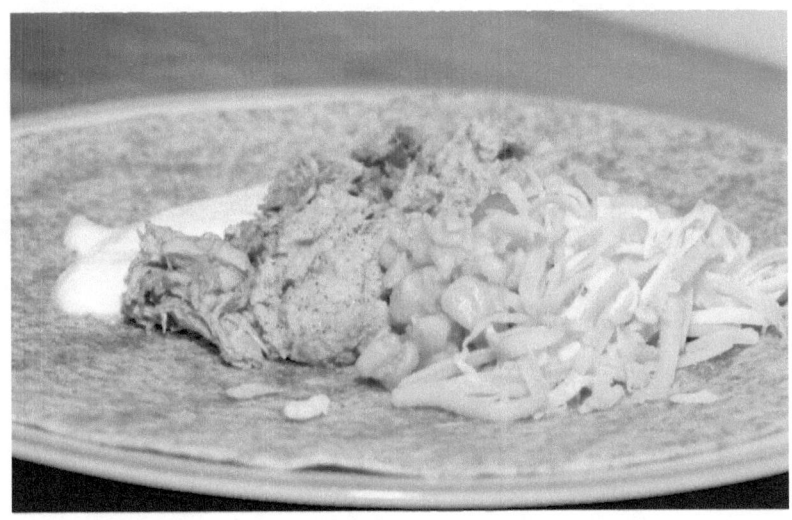

At a kick to your gout friendly menu by adding some salsa chicken burritos in the mix.

Yield: 4

Preparation Time: 35 minutes

Ingredient List:

- chicken breast (2 pieces, bone lessons skinless, halved)
- tomato sauce (4 ounces)
- salsa (¼ cup)
- taco seasoning (1.25 ounces)
- cumin (1 teaspoon, ground)
- garlic (2 cloves, minced)
- chili powder (1 teaspoon)
- Hot sauce (2 tablespoons)

HHHHHHHHHHHHHHHHHHHHHHHHHHHHHHHHH

Instructions:

1. Allow your chicken breasts to come to a boil with your tomato sauce over medium heat in a saucepan.

2. Once boiling, add any remaining ingredients and allow to simmer for at least 15 minutes.

3. Using a fork, pull your chicken into thin strings then return to the pot, cover and cook for at least 10 more minutes. Enjoy!

Recipe 11: Cherry, Banana & Strawberry Smoothie

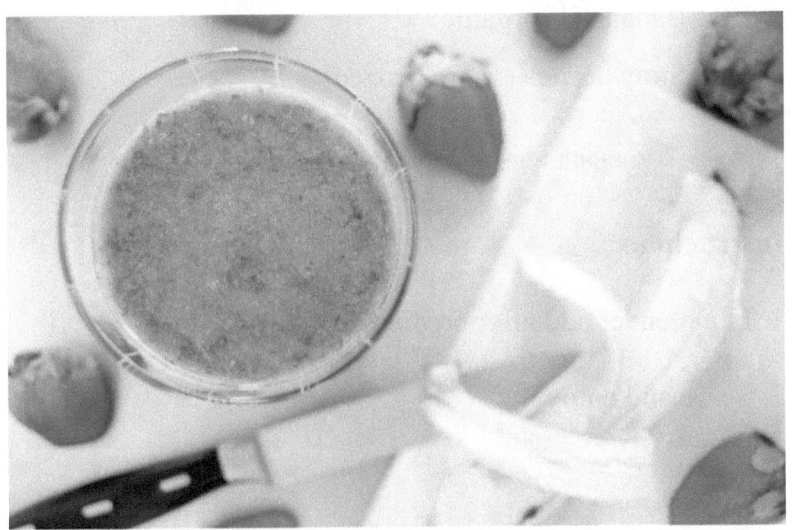

When you have gout it's important to stick to foods that provide you with the necessary anthocyanins to help relieve you of inflammation. Here is a recipe that will help you accomplish that.

Yield: 2

Preparation Time: 15 minutes.

Ingredient List:

- 2 cup cherries, frozen
- 1 ½ cup almond milk
- Banana (1, organic)
- Strawberries (1 cup, frozen)

HHHHHHHHHHHHHHHHHHHHHHHHHHHHHHHH

Instructions:

1. In a blender add all ingredients and blend well.

2. Serve and enjoy.

Recipe 12: Lemon Dill Salmon

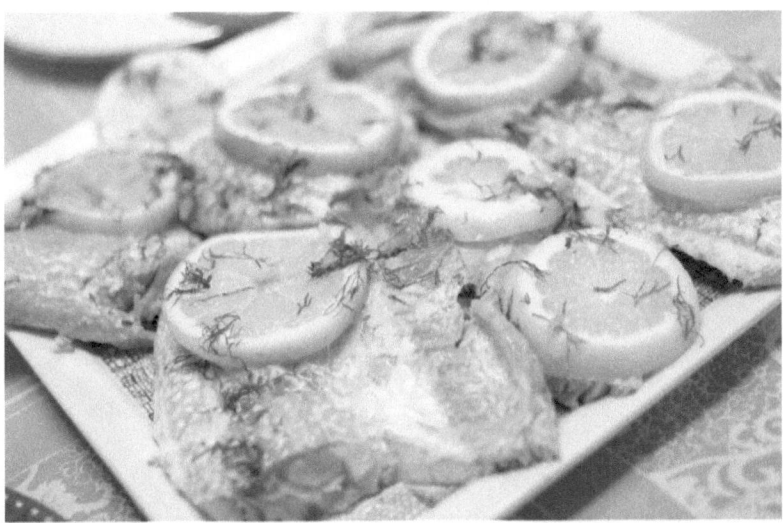

Selecting good gout friendly lunch can be difficult. Enjoy this delicious salmon dish knowing that it's not only gout friendly but delicious.

Yield: 4

Preparation Time: 35 minutes

Ingredient List:

- salmon (1 pound, fillets)
- butter (¼ cup, melted)
- dill weed (1 tablespoon)
- Garlic powder (¼ teaspoons)
- Sea salt (1 teaspoon)
- Black pepper (1 teaspoon)

HHHHHHHHHHHHHHHHHHHHHHHHHHHHHHHHHH

Instructions:

1. Set your oven to preheat to 350° F and prepare a baking dish by lightly greasing.

2. Adding the salmon into the prepared baking this and drizzle your remaining ingredients on top.

3. Set to bake until salmon is fully cooked (about 25 minutes). Enjoy!

Recipe 13: Brown Stewed Chicken

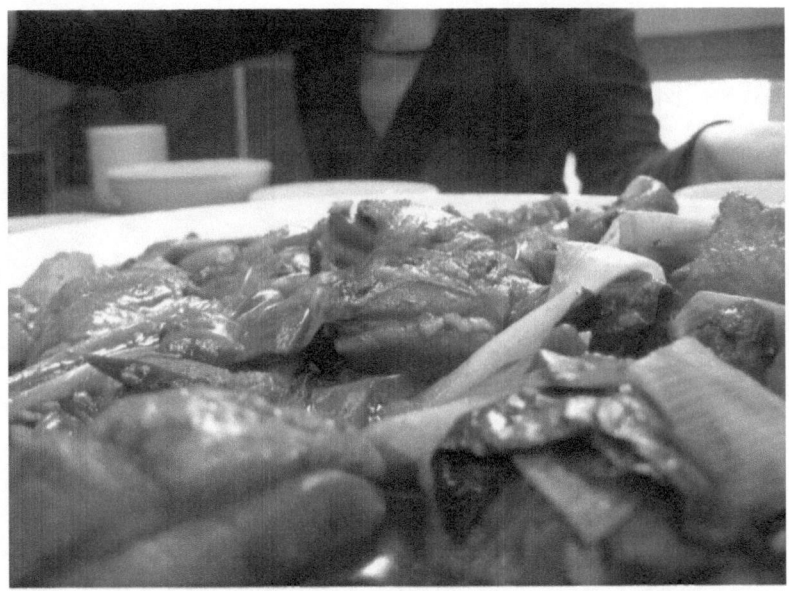

If soul-warming food is your cup of tea, then you need to try out this recipe.

Yield: 6

Preparation Time: 4 hours 15 minutes

Ingredient List:

- 3lbs chicken, sectioned
- 1 tablespoon Worcestershire sauce
- 14oz. can coconut milk
- ½ cup chicken stock
- 2 tablespoons fish sauce
- 2 tablespoons brown sugar
- 2 teaspoons browning
- 1 tablespoon lemon juice
- 2 limes, juiced and zested
- 1 tablespoon olive oil
- ½ teaspoon Salt
- ¼ teaspoon Pepper

HHHHHHHHHHHHHHHHHHHHHHHHHHHHHHHH

Instructions:

1. Heat the oil in a dutch oven over medium-high heat. Season the chicken and cook in the oil until browned on all sides.

2. Add the Worcestershire sauce, brown sugar, and lemon juice. Cook until the sugar is melted.

3. Next, add in your remaining ingredients, cover and cook on high for 30 – 45 minutes.

Recipe 14: Potato and Vegetable Frittata

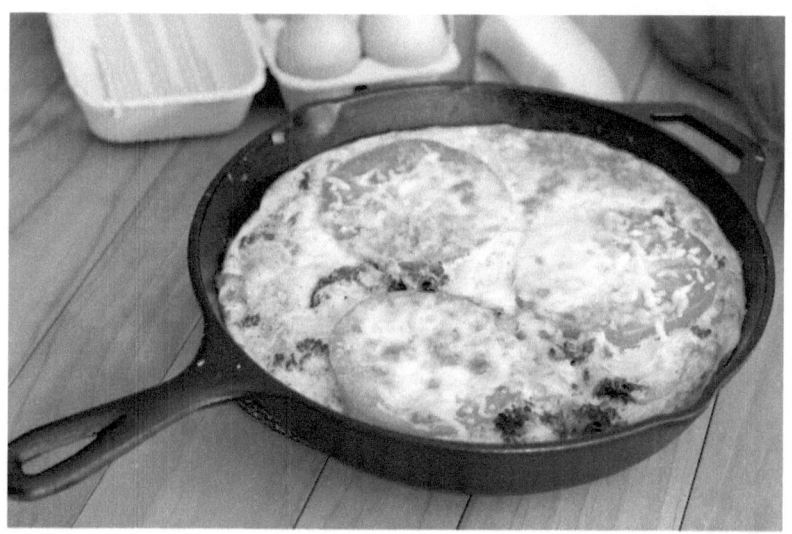

Here we have a delicious breakfast option for your gout friendly menu.

Yield: 2

Preparation Time: 25 minutes

Ingredient List:

- olive oil (1 teaspoon)
- Onion (½ cup, chopped)
- garlic (1 clove, minced)
- Bell Pepper (½ cup, diced, green)
- zucchini (1, cut into ¼ inch matchsticks)
- potatoes (2 cups, cooked, diced)
- tomato (1 cup, chopped)
- olives (2 tablespoons, Black)
- eggs (4, large)
- salt (1 teaspoon)
- black pepper (1 teaspoon)
- Oregano (¼ teaspoons)
- Cayenne pepper (¼ teaspoons)
- Cherry tomato (½, small, sliced)
- mozzarella (¼ cup, shredded)
- Parmesan cheese (¼ cup, grated)

HHHHHHHHHHHHHHHHHHHHHHHHHHHHHHHHH

Instructions:

1. Set your boiler to preheat to high.

2. Sauté your bell pepper, garlic, and onion with oil in an ovenproof skillet until tender.

3. Add your potatoes, and stir to combine.

4. Next, add your zucchini, tomatoes, and olives, and continue to stir until potatoes have become tender.

5. In a separate bowl, combine your egg and seasoning (cayenne pepper, black pepper, salt, and oregano) and whisk to combine.

6. Pour your eggs over your vegetable mixture in your skillet, arrange or cherry tomatoes on top of the eggs, top with cheeses, and allow to cook until eggs are almost set.

7. Place your skillet under your boiler until eggs have been fully set, and cheeses form a nice golden-brown crust. Serve and enjoy!

Recipe 15: Creamy Peanut Soup

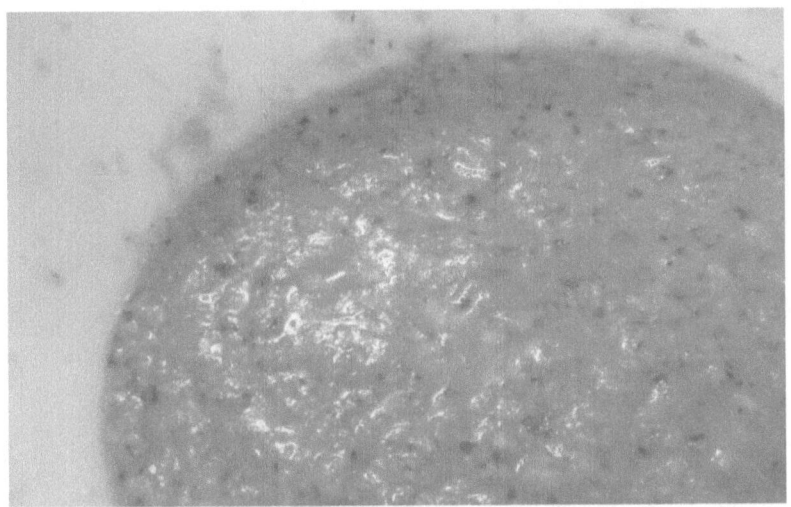

This bowl of soup will wow you!

Yield: 8

Preparation Time: 4 hours 10 minutes

Ingredient List:

- 4lb. skinless and boneless chicken breasts
- 2 tablespoons lime juice
- 4 cups chicken broth
- 4 tablespoon honey
- 1 cup peanut butter, preferably chunky
- 2 green bell peppers sliced
- 2 brown onions, diced
- 2 red bell peppers, sliced
- ½ cup soy sauce
- ½ cup crushed peanuts, for topping

HHHHHHHHHHHHHHHHHHHHHHHHHHHHHHHH

Instructions:

1. Place the sliced bell peppers and diced onion in the bottom of slow cooker.

2. In a medium bowl, whisk the peanut butter, soy sauce, lime juice, honey, and chicken broth.

3. Cook on high for 30 minutes then transfer your soup to either a blender or food processor and pulse until smooth.

4. Sprinkle with peanuts, serve, and enjoy.

Recipe 16: Honey Mustard Chicken

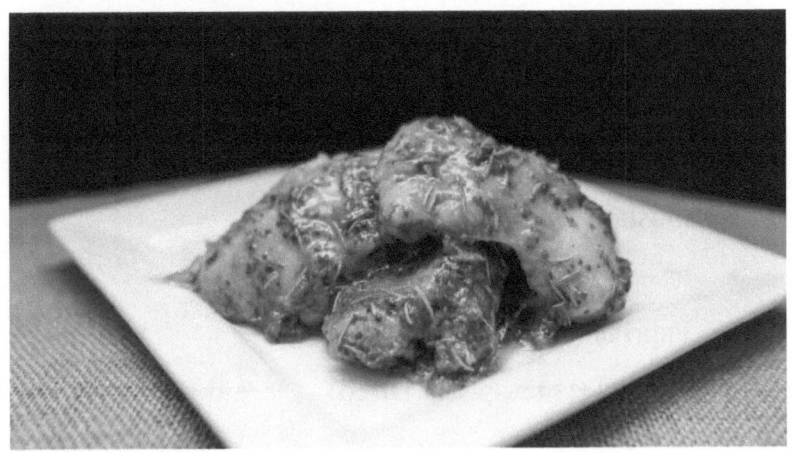

Here is a delicious gout friendly recipe that the whole family can enjoy.

Yield: 6

Preparation Time: 1 hour

Ingredient List:

- chicken breasts (6 pieces, boneless and skinless)
- salt (½ teaspoon)
- Black pepper (½ teaspoon)
- Honey (½ cup)
- mustard (½ cup, Dijon)
- basil (1 teaspoon)
- Paprika (1 teaspoon)
- Parsley (½ teaspoon, Dried)

HHHHHHHHHHHHHHHHHHHHHHHHHHHHHHHH

Instructions:

1. Set your oven to preheat to 350° F, and prepare a baking dish by lightly greasing.

2. Season your chicken breasts by sprinkling with your salt and pepper.

3. Combine your remaining ingredients in a small bowl and mix well.

4. Brush a half of this mixture over chicken, and placed to bake for 30 minutes.

5. Turn the chicken pieces over, brush with your remaining honey mustard glaze, and allow to cook for another 15 minutes. Remove from heat and serve.

Recipe 17: Lentil Soup

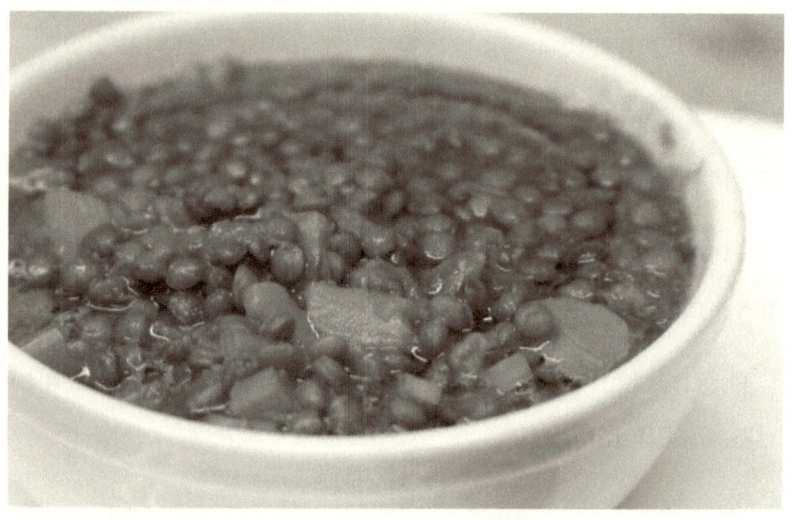

Enjoy this warm bowl of soup on a cold winter day.

Yield: 4

Preparation Time: 1 hour

Ingredient List:

- 1 cup brown lentils
- 4 cups vegetable broth
- ½ bay leaf
- ¼ teaspoon ground coriander seeds
- ½ tablespoon olive oil
- ½ teaspoon Salt
- ¼ teaspoon Pepper

HHHHHHHHHHHHHHHHHHHHHHHHHHHHHHHH

Instructions:

1. Rinse the lentils under cold water and remove any black ones.

2. Place the rinsed lentils into a rice cooker.

3. Add the remaining ingredients and give it a good stir.

4. Cover and cook for 60 minutes.

5. Season to taste and serve while still hot.

Recipe 18: Vanilla Fruit Salad

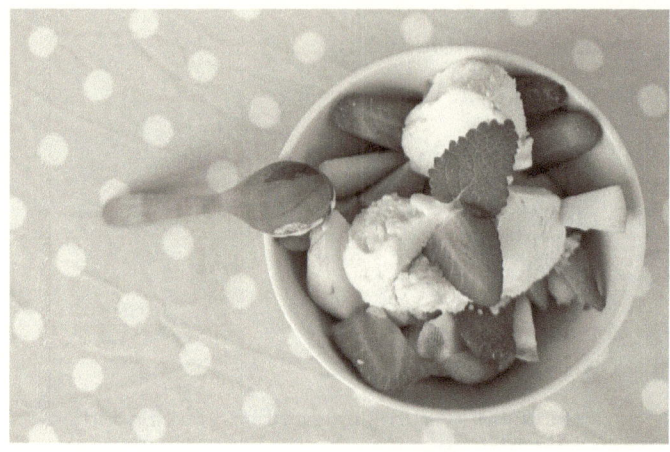

If you like sweet breakfast dishes, then this is a must try. This dish is filled with nutrients and antioxidants to help ease gout pain.

Yield: 6

Preparation Time: 15 minutes

Ingredient List:

- Apples (2 cups, diced)
- banana (1 cup, sliced)
- strawberries (1 cup, sliced, fresh)
- walnuts (1 cup, chopped)
- yogurt (1 cup, vanilla)
- cinnamon (¾ teaspoons, Ground)

HHHHHHHHHHHHHHHHHHHHHHHHHHHHHHHH

Instructions:

1. Combine all your ingredients in a large bowl, stir gently. Serve and enjoy!

Recipe 19: Spicy Pan-Fried Chicken

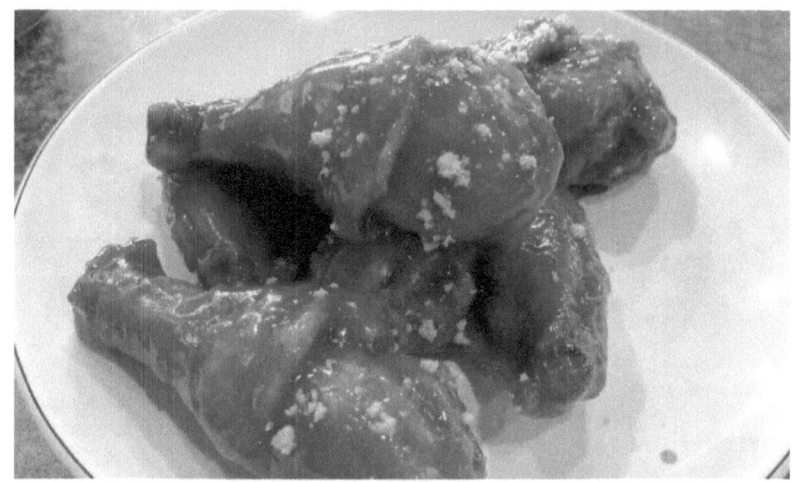

If you like spice then this is a tasty gout friendly recipe that will please your palate.

Serve: 3

Preparation Time: 30 minutes

Ingredient List:

- Chopped onion: ¼ cup
- Soy sauce: 5 tablespoons
- Minced garlic: 2 tablespoons
- Brown sugar: 2 ½ tablespoons
- Sesame oil: 2 tablespoons
- Sesame seeds: 1 tablespoon
- Cayenne: ½ tsp
- Salt and pepper
- Boneless chicken breasts, strips: 1 lb.

HHHHHHHHHHHHHHHHHHHHHHHHHHHHHHH

Instructions:

1. Take a bowl and mix all ingredients except chicken.

2. Put chicken in mixture and coat well.

3. Take a skillet and transfer mixture with chicken into it.

4. Cook on a medium heat for 20 minutes.

5. Serve, and enjoy.

Recipe 20: Slow Cooker Chicken Stew

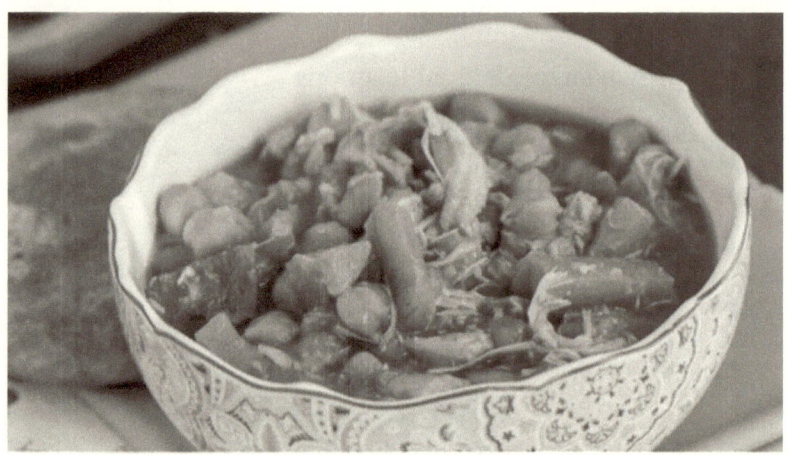

Consuming too much red meat is taboo for gout patients. This doesn't mean, however, that you can't enjoy a delicious stew.

Yield: 6

Preparation Time: 4 hours

Ingredient List:

- chicken thigh (2 lbs., cut into small pieces)
- flour (¼ cup, all-purpose)
- salt (½ teaspoons)
- Black pepper (½ teaspoons)
- Garlic (1 clove, minced)
- bay leaf (1)
- paprika (1 teaspoon)
- Worcestershire sauce (1 teaspoon)
- Onion (1, chopped)
- beef broth (1 ½ cups)
- potatoes (3, diced)
- carrots (4, sliced)
- celery (1 stalk, chopped)

HHHHHHHHHHHHHHHHHHHHHHHHHHHHHHH

Instructions:

1. Combine all your ingredients in a slow cooker, cover, and allow to cook on high for about 4 hours. Serve and enjoy!

Recipe 21: Hoisin Chicken Filled Lettuce Wraps

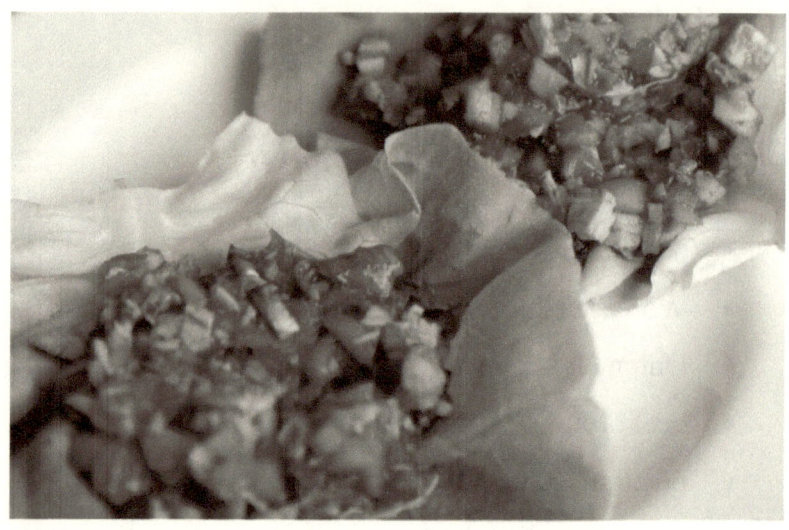

These wraps are typically a popular item in bars, and now you can enjoy them from your kitchen.

Yield: 4

Preparation Time: 25 minutes

Ingredient List:

- Chicken breasts (12 oz., sliced)
- Olive oil (2 teaspoons)
- Onion (1, chopped)
- Black pepper (¼ teaspoon)
- Butter Lettuce (12 leaves, washed and separated)
- Garlic (2 cloves, minced)
- Ginger Powder (½ teaspoon)
- Hoisin sauce (3 tablespoons)
- Sesame Seeds (1/8 cup, black, and white)

HHHHHHHHHHHHHHHHHHHHHHHHHHHHHHHHH

Instructions:

1. Set oven to 350°F.

2. Heat half of the oil in a skillet and add onion, and garlic then cook for about 3 minutes.

3. Add your chicken, and toss to combine. Add in your hoisin sauce, stir to combine, and place in oven to cook until done (about 10 minutes).

4. Spoon chicken mixture into butter lettuce leaves.

5. Serve, and enjoy.

Recipe 22: Cherry Smoothie

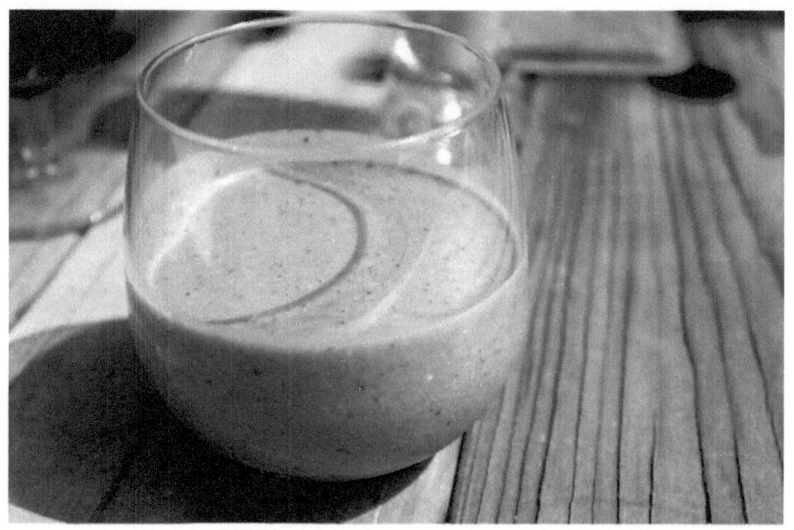

Cherries are known to help decrease inflammation levels in the body making it great for gout patients.

Yield: 2

Preparation Time: 15 minutes

Ingredient List:

- 2 cup cherries, frozen
- 1 cup almond milk
- ½ cup coconut milk
- Few ice chunks (about 6)

HHHHHHHHHHHHHHHHHHHHHHHHHHHHHHHHH

Instructions:

1. In a blender add all ingredients and blend well.

2. Serve and enjoy.

Recipe 23: Sweet & Spicy Chicken Wings

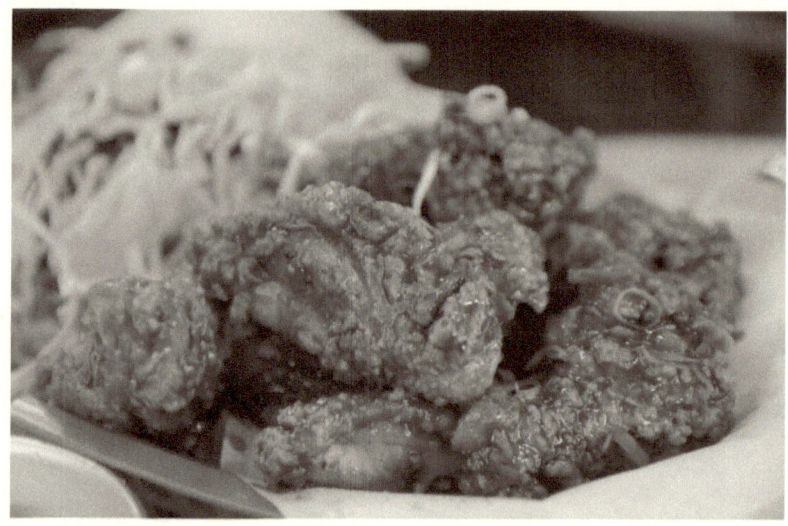

Chicken wings are thankfully fair game, even with gout.

Servings: 4

Preparation Time: 1 hour 30 minutes

Ingredient List:

- Chicken Wings (3 lbs.)
- Extra Virgin Coconut Oil (2 tablespoons)
- Garlic (4 cloves, chopped)
- Ginger (1 tablespoon, chopped)
- Siracha Sauce (3 tablespoons)
- Coconut Aminos (½ cup)
- Sherry (2 tablespoons)
- Honey (2 tablespoons)
- Apple Cider Vinegar (2 tablespoons)
- Fish Sauce (1 tablespoon)
- Peanut Oil (2 tablespoons)
- Salt (2 teaspoons)
- Black Pepper (1 teaspoon)
- Cajun spice (2 teaspoons)

HHHHHHHHHHHHHHHHHHHHHHHHHHHHHHHH

Instructions:

1. Put wings into a large bowl, drain or pat to dry. Season well with salt, Cajun spice, and pepper, then set aside

2. In a small saucepan heat oil then add garlic, and ginger. Add all your remaining, and stir to create a sweet and spicy wing sauce. Remove from flame and add sesame oil.

3. Bake wings at 375 °until they are done.

4. Pour sauce mixture over wings and toss to coat.

5. Serve and enjoy!

Recipe 24: Mushroom & Chicken Stuffed Bell Peppers

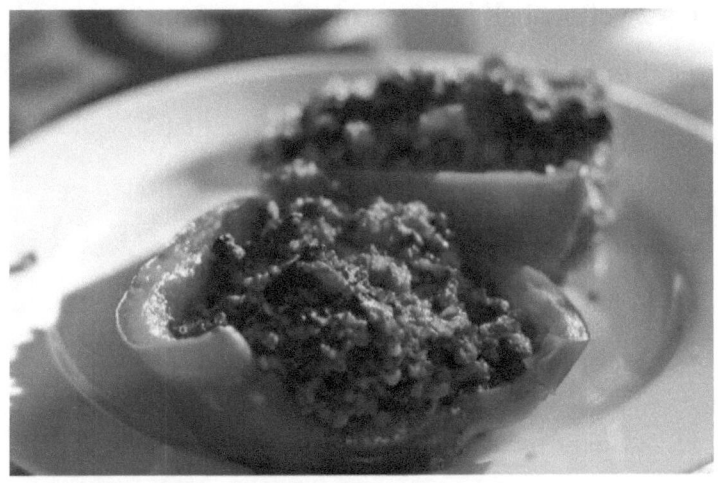

Here's a delicious dinner option that is fit for the whole family.

Yield: 4

Preparation Time: 35 minutes

Ingredient List:

- 1 cup Portobello mushrooms, chopped
- 2 red bell peppers, make a cut from stem
- 2 yellow bell peppers, make a cut from stem
- 1 cup chicken mince
- ½ cup tomato puree
- ¼ teaspoon garlic paste
- ½ teaspoon black pepper
- ¼ teaspoon salt
- 2 tablespoons olive oil

HHHHHHHHHHHHHHHHHHHHHHHHHHHHHHH

Instructions:

1. Heat oil in a pan and add garlic, fry for 1 minute.

2. Add chicken mince and mushrooms, then stir well.

3. When chicken mince becomes golden brown add tomato puree and fry again for 5-10 minutes.

4. Season with salt and pepper.

5. Preheat oven to 355 degrees.

6. Fill bell peppers with fried mince and place into greased pan.

7. Bake for 10 minutes.

8. Serve and enjoy.

Recipe 25: Grilled Chicken & Green Bean Salad

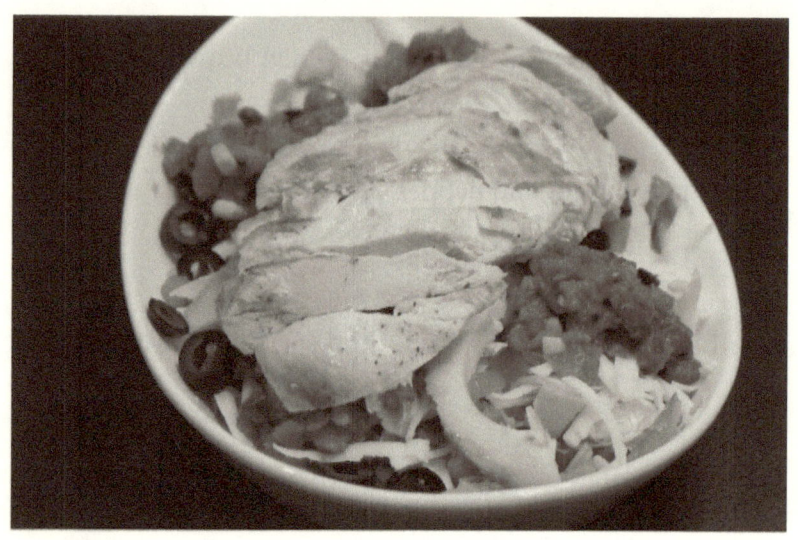

This salad is heaven to all chicken lovers.

Yield: 4

Preparation Time: 15 minutes

Ingredient List:

- Haricot Verts (¼ cup, blanched and chopped into halves)
- Basil (½ cup, chopped)
- Chicken (1 lbs., grilled, sliced)
- Olive Oil (4 tablespoons)
- Garlic (2 cloves, crushed)
- Salt (¾ tsp)
- Vinegar (2 tablespoons)
- Pepper (½ teaspoons)

HHHHHHHHHHHHHHHHHHHHHHHHHHHHHHH

Instructions:

1. In a small bowl, create a dressing by whipping together your vinegar, olive oil, garlic, salt, and pepper.

2. In another bowl add your remaining ingredients then pour the dressing over it.

3. Toss until evenly coated.

4. Serve and enjoy!

Recipe 26: Chicken Mince Salad

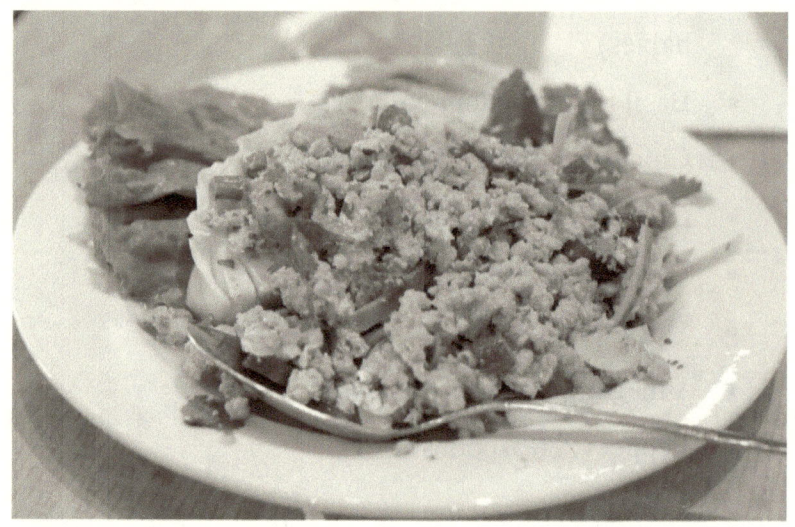

This delicious salad will keep you fuller longer.

Serves 4

Preparation Time: 35 minutes

Ingredient List:

- 1 oz. minced chicken
- Mint (1/3 cup)
- 1 onion, chopped
- 1 head baby cos lettuce, washed and separated
- 1 cup tomato puree
- ¼ teaspoon garlic paste
- ½ teaspoon chili powder
- ¼ teaspoon turmeric powder
- 1 bunch fresh coriander, chopped
- 1 lemon
- 2 green chilies
- ½ teaspoon cumin powder
- ½ teaspoon cinnamon powder
- 2 cups chicken broth
- ¼ teaspoon salt
- 2 tablespoons olive oil

HHHHHHHHHHHHHHHHHHHHHHHHHHHHHHHHH

Instructions:

1. Heat oil in a pan and add onion, fry for 2 minutes.

2. Add chicken mince with garlic and fry well until nicely golden.

3. Add tomato puree and fry again for 5-10 minutes.

4. Add salt, chili powder, turmeric powder. Stir.

5. Add remaining ingredients, and cover with lid. Leave to cook on low heat for 15 minutes.

6. Transfer lettuce onto a serving dish and top chicken mince.

7. Squeeze lemon juice.

8. Serve and enjoy.

Recipe 27: Garlic Mashed Red Potato

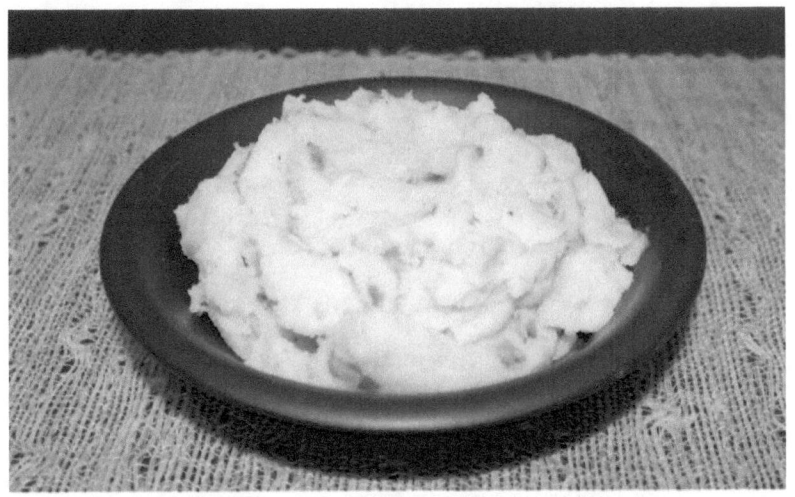

Enjoy this hearty mash as a delicious side dish.

Yield: 4

Preparation Time: 30 minutes

Ingredient List:

- Red Potatoes (2 cups, diced, cooked)
- Garlic (8 cloves, crushed)
- Olive Oil (6 tablespoons)
- Butter (½ cup, unsalted)
- Salt (1 teaspoon)
- Pepper (¾ teaspoon)
- Green Onions (1 stalk, diced)
- Radishes (4, medium, sliced)
- Carrot (1 medium, diced)
- Sweet Pepper (1 medium, diced)

HHHHHHHHHHHHHHHHHHHHHHHHHHHHHHHH

Instructions:

1. In a large bowl, thoroughly combine all your ingredients until fully incorporated.

2. Mash with a potato masher, serve and enjoy.

Recipe 28: Roasted Carrot & Bell Pepper Soup

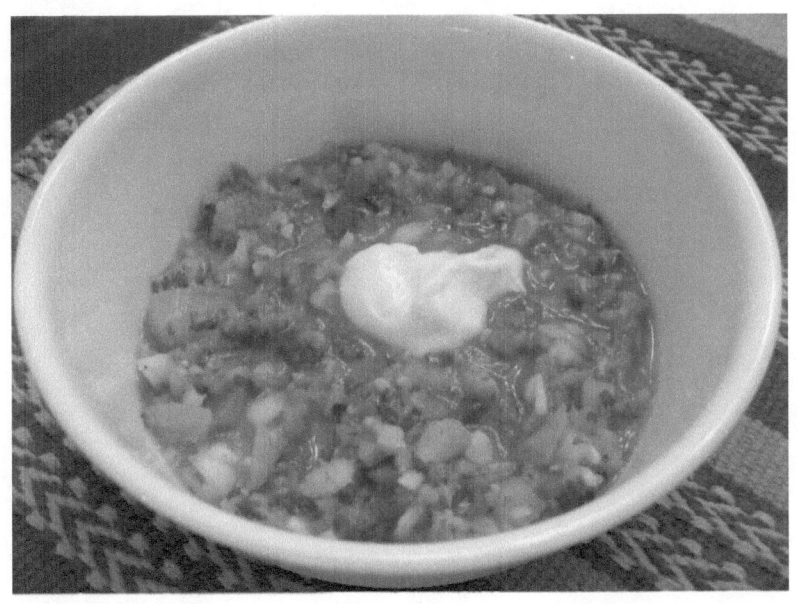

Enjoy this bowl of low cholesterol vegetable soup.

Yield: 5

Preparation Time: 35 minutes

Ingredient List:

- Extra Virgin Olive Oil (2 teaspoons)
- Shallots (½ cup, chopped)
- Bell Pepper (3 cups, roasted, peeled, cubed)
- Carrots (1½ cup, peeled, roasted, chopped)
- Ginger (1 tablespoon, grated)
- Chicken broth (3 cups, fat-free)
- Salt (¼ teaspoons)

HHHHHHHHHHHHHHHHHHHHHHHHHHHHHHHHHH

Instructions:

1. Place a saucepan with your oil on medium heat until it just begins to smoke.

2. Add your shallots to the pot and sauté until it becomes tender (should take approximately 2 – 3 min).

3. Add the shallots all your prepped vegetables then allow to cook for another 2 minutes.

4. Pour in your broth and allow it to come to a boil. Once boiling, place the lid on the pot and reduce the heat to low.

5. Allow this mixture to simmer until your vegetables are all tender. Once tender, add salt and pour your soup into a food processor.

6. Pulse until creamy and smooth. Serve and Enjoy.

Recipe 29: Sunomono Salad

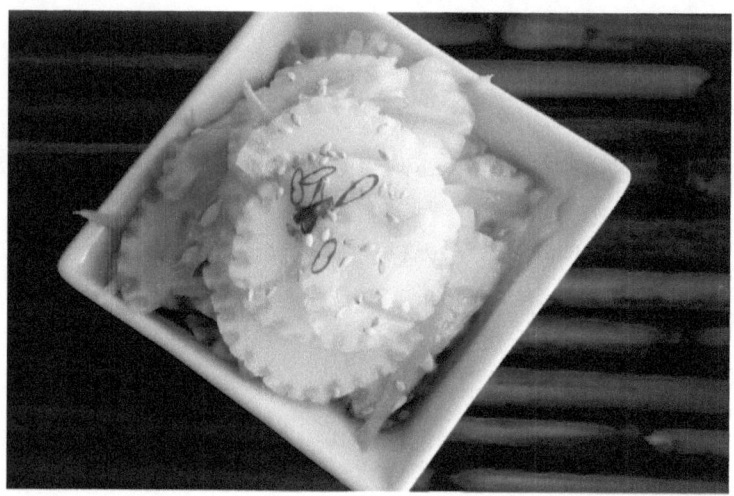

This salad is simple to make and creates the perfect snack.

Yield: 4 – 6

Preparation Time: 10 minutes

Ingredient List:

- Cucumber (1 English, thinly sliced)
- Rice Vinegar (½ cup)
- Sugar (2 tablespoons)
- Coriander Seeds (2 teaspoons, toasted)
- Salt (½ teaspoons)
- Red Pepper Flakes (¼ teaspoons)

HHHHHHHHHHHHHHHHHHHHHHHHHHHHHHHH

Instructions:

1. In a medium-sized serving bowl thorough mix all the ingredients together until well incorporated minutes. Serve and enjoy!

Recipe 30: Sweet & Nutty Fruit Salad

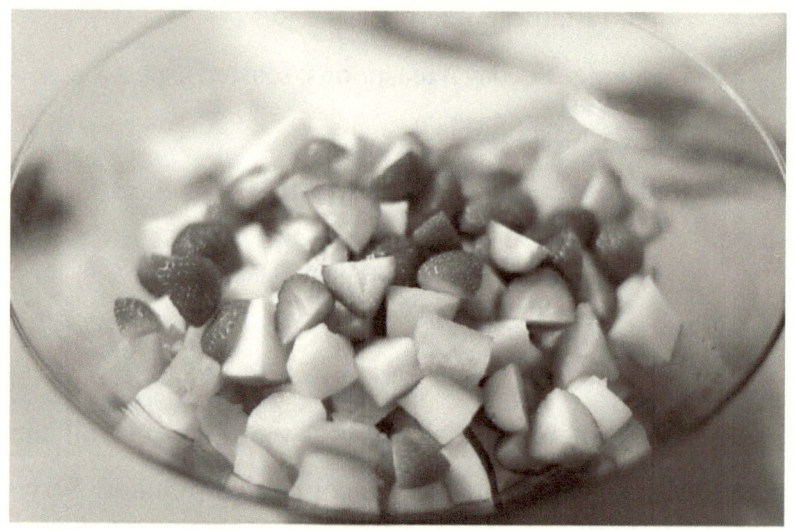

Here is a salad that even the kids will love.

Yield: 4

Preparation Time: 5 min

Ingredient List:

- Mayonnaise (2 tablespoons, low-fat)
- Lemon Juice (1 tablespoon)
- Apples (2 Granny Smith, small, cubed)
- Grapes (1 cup, red, halves)
- Cherries (1/3 cup, dried)
- Almonds (¼ cup, chopped)
- Grapes (¼ cup, sliced)

HHHHHHHHHHHHHHHHHHHHHHHHHHHHHHH

Instructions:

1. Create a dressing in a medium bowl by whipping the lemon juice and mayonnaise until fully combined.

2. Add your fruits, and almonds to the dressing and mix until fully coated.

3. Serve, and enjoy.

About the Author

Angel Burns learned to cook when she worked in the local seafood restaurant near her home in Hyannis Port in Massachusetts as a teenager. The head chef took Angel under his wing and taught the young woman the tricks of the trade for cooking seafood. The skills she had learned at a young age helped her get accepted into Boston University's Culinary Program where she also minored in business administration.

Summers off from school meant working at the same restaurant but when Angel's mentor and friend retired as head chef, she took over after graduation and created classic and new dishes that delighted the diners. The restaurant flourished under Angel's culinary creativity and one customer developed more than an appreciation for Angel's food. Several months after taking over the position, the young woman met her future husband at work and they have been inseparable ever since. They still live in Hyannis Port with their two children and a cocker spaniel named Buddy.

Angel Burns turned her passion for cooking and her business acumen into a thriving e-book business. She has authored several successful books on cooking different types of dishes using simple ingredients for novices and experienced chefs alike. She is still head chef in Hyannis Port and says she will probably never leave!

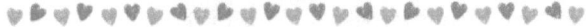

Author's Afterthoughts

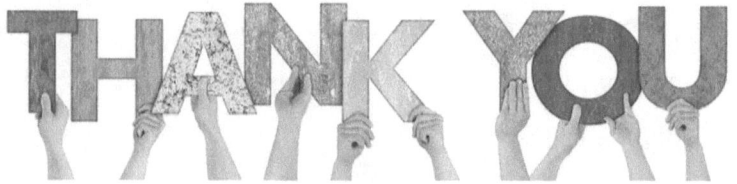

With so many books out there to choose from, I want to thank you for choosing this one and taking precious time out of your life to buy and read my work. Readers like you are the reason I take such passion in creating these books.

It is with gratitude and humility that I express how honored I am to become a part of your life and I hope that you take the same pleasure in reading this book as I did in writing it.

Can I ask one small favour? I ask that you write an honest and open review on Amazon of what you thought of the book. This will help other readers make an informed choice on whether to buy this book.

My sincerest thanks,

Angel Burns

If you want to be the first to know about news, new books, events and giveaways, subscribe to my newsletter by clicking the link below

https://angel-burns.gr8.com

or Scan QR-code

www.ingramcontent.com/pod-product-compliance
Lightning Source LLC
Chambersburg PA
CBHW022130170526
45157CB00004B/1816